USMLE STEP 2 CK
Gastroenterology
In Your Pocket

✓ Study guide for the USMLE STEP 2 CK exam.

✓ Prepare for your shelf examination.

✓ Be ready for your inpatient rotation.

Gregory J. Fernandez M.D.

This book is gratefully dedicated to my wife. Thank you for your support and always being there for me. Thank you for your kindness, your devotion, and your endless selflessness support. I love you... Thank you mother, father, step-mother, brothers, friends, and family for all your encouragement and endless love. Best of luck to all the medical dreamers, the road is long and I hope my book helps you through this journey. All the best...

First Edition, 2016

Author & Editor: Gregory J. Fernandez, M.D.

Publisher: M.D. Educational Services

Peer-reviewer: Dr. Arslan Talat, M.D. Services, Institute of Medical Sciences, Pakistand

Cover Desing: Dustin Williams & Marie Meyer

Book Design: Marie Meyer

Copyediting: Editage Cactus Communications

DISCLAIMER: The author, editor, publisher, and staff members have taken care to confirm the accuracy of the information present in this publication. The context of the books entirety, is believed to be reliable in accordance with the standards accepted at the time of publication. However, readers are encouraged to confirm the information and conduct their own research for clarification of all the information present within this book. No one involved in creating this book is responsible for errors or omissions or for any consequences from application of the information in this book. There is no warranty, expressed or implied, with respect to the completeness or accuracy of the contents of this publication. Neither the editor, nor the author assumes any liability for any injury and/or damage to persons or property arising from the content of this publication. Application of this information in a particular situation remains the professional responsibility of the practitioner; the clinical treatments or information described and recommended may not be considered absolute and universal recommendations. It is the responsibility of the health care provider to ascertain the FDA status of each drug used or device planned for use in their clinical practice. The purpose of this books, is to be used as a study guide for medical examinations. Please consult with attending physicians for any medical decisions.

ISBN-13: 978-1530130894

ISBN-10: 1530130891

How to Use
"Gastroenterology In Your Pocket"

Gastroenterology In Your Pocket is a study guide for the USMLE STEP 2 CK exam that you can also use to prepare for your shelf examination and to get ready for your inpatient rotation. It is part of a series, each dealing with a different subject or sub-specialty, focusing on vital clinical knowledge.

The subjects and topics within gastroenterology are called out in large, colored type. These items are also included in the Table of Contents for ease of access.

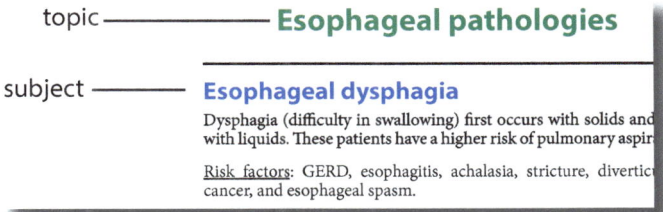

Many subjects also contain sub-subjects that are also called out in bold, blue type either as bulleted items or in-line with the text, as

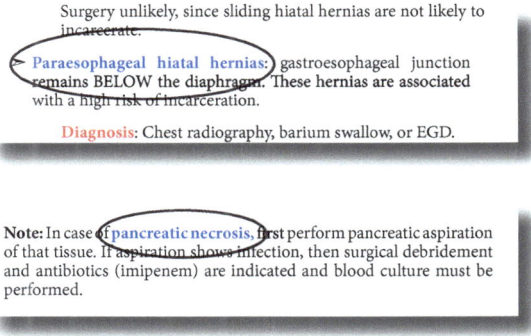

Presentation of clinical history and physical exam (Hx/PE), step-by-step diagnosis, and treatment plan are indicated by bold red headings.

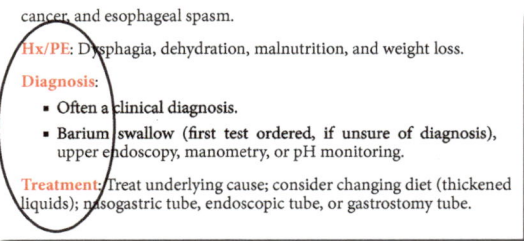

Procedures, triads, pathology, medications, antibodies and findings are called out in bold text. These items are also included in the index.

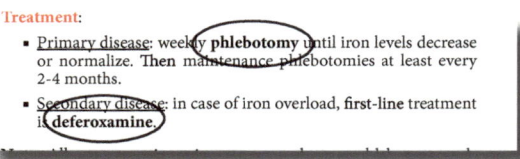

Reflexes, signs and maneuvers are shown in purple text.

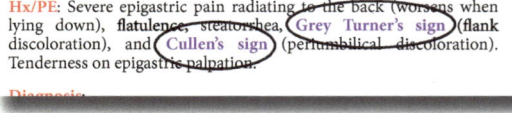

Mnemonics and key words are shown in orange text.

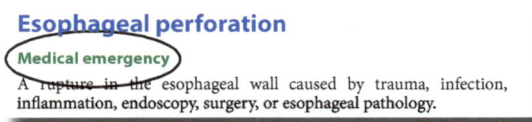

And, finally, for the avoidance of doubt, circumstances that amount to a medical emergency are flagged with warning.

Esophageal perforation

Medical emergency

A rupture in the esophageal wall caused by trauma, infection, inflammation, endoscopy, surgery, or esophageal pathology.

Gastroenterology
Table of Contents

Esophageal pathologies

Esophageal dysphagia

Dysphagia (difficulty in swallowing) first occurs with solids and then with liquids. These patients have a higher risk of pulmonary aspiration.

<u>Risk factors</u>: GERD, esophagitis, achalasia, stricture, diverticulum, cancer, and esophageal spasm.

Hx/PE: Dysphagia, dehydration, malnutrition, and weight loss.

Diagnosis:
- Often a clinical diagnosis.
- Barium swallow (first test ordered, if unsure of diagnosis), upper endoscopy, manometry, or pH monitoring.

Treatment: Treat underlying cause; consider changing diet (thickened liquids); nasogastric tube, endoscopic tube, or gastrostomy tube.

Note: Provide aspiration pneumonia prevention--Sit in an upright position when eating food or drinking fluids, diet considerations, and small frequent meals.

Oropharyngeal dysphagia

Occurs when initiating the <u>involuntary</u> process of swallowing (moving food from the mouth to the throat). Usually associated with neuromuscular disorders such as, multiple sclerosis, scleroderma, dementia, stroke, or Parkinson's disease.

Hx/PE: Weight loss, malnutrition, dehydration, and frequent episodes of aspiration pneumonia.

Diagnosis: Mini mental state examination (MMSE), swallow study, barium swallow, and endoscopy.

Treatment:
- Treat underlying cause; will often need to change diet to thickened liquids.
- Swallowing techniques such as eating with head back and neck

extended. There are many techniques depending on what works best for the patient.

Note: May need to consider nasogastric feeding tube or gastrostomy tube placement.

Esophageal webs (Plummer-Vinson syndrome)

Associated with iron-deficiency anemia and glossitis. Increased risk of developing squamous cell carcinoma of the esophagus.

Hx/PE: Dysphagia (solids > liquids), acid reflux, cheilosis, and fatigue.

Diagnosis:

- CBC (anemia), MCV (low), and iron studies (low iron levels with elevated TIBC).
- Barium swallow and endoscopy ("**webs and strictures**").

Treatment:

- First, control acid reflux (PPIs) and start iron supplementation.
- If iron supplementation is not helpful, esophageal balloon dilation will be necessary to break-up the esophageal webs.

Esophagitis

Inflammation of the esophagus that can be acute or chronic. Commonly secondary to GERD, infections (CMV, candida), alcohol abuse, intubated patients, or chronic medication use (especially potassium and bisphosphonate supplementation).

Hx/PE: Burning sensation in the esophagus and dry cough, especially in the morning.

Diagnosis: Upper endoscopy with biopsy, tests followed will depend on what endoscopy reveals.

Treatment:

- Treat underlying cause.
- Keep in mind, in HIV patients need to consider esophageal candidiasis (treat with oral fluconazole).

Note: If esophagitis caused by medications, take while sitting up (remain seated for at least 30 minutes) and drink plenty of water.

Nutcracker esophagus

An abnormally high-pressure contraction of the smooth muscles of the esophagus.

Hx/PE: Very similar presentation to diffuse esophageal spasm. Patients present with upper chest discomfort and pressure.

Diagnosis: Barium swallow and esophageal manometry (**esophageal motility study**) distal peristaltic amplitudes are >180 mmHg [most specific diagnostic study]).

Treatment: Calcium channel blockers (**diltiazem**). Use peripheral specific blockers and avoid cardiac-specific calcium channel blockers. Nitrates can also be useful.

Note: If diagnosis is unclear need to rule out other causes of chest pain such as myocardial infarction, pancreatitis, GERD, costochondritis, and peptic ulcers.

Esophageal spasm

Intermittent painful muscle contractions that clinically mimic acute myocardial infarction (**Prinzmetal's angina**). Dysphagia more common with solids and less with liquids. Can be triggered by drinking cold or hot beverages.

Diagnosis:

- Barium swallow, in case of active episode of spasm (may show "corkscrew" appearance).
- Esophageal manometry (most accurate): high-intensity "disorganized contractions."

Treatment: Calcium-channel blockers (peripheral-specific, like diltiazem) and dietary lifestyle modification. Nitrates can also be useful.

Note:
✓ Need to rule out MI with EKG and troponin levels.

✓ The treatment for esophageal spasm is similar, as for that of Prinzmetal's angina.

Vascular rings (peptic strictures)

Tracheal compression, caused by esophageal scarring, fibrosis, and strictures. Dysphagia mainly with solids followed by liquids. Gradual luminal narrowing usually secondary to chronic gastroesophageal reflux.

Hx/PE: Painless dysphagia (often intermediate), choking, difficulty swallowing, and acid reflux.

Diagnosis: Barium swallow and upper endoscopy; both showing "ring-like structures."

Treatment:

- Aggressive anti-reflux medication (first-line treatment) and endoscopic dilation (in severe cases).
- Surgery is needed if symptomatic and not controlled by other methods.

Esophageal diverticula

Considered a false diverticula; does not include outpouching of all the layers.

➤ Zenker's diverticulum: above the upper esophageal sphincter.

➤ Traction diverticulum: mid-esophagus.

➤ Epiphrenic diverticulum: above the lower esophageal sphincter.

Hx/PE: Dysphagia, chest pain, "halitosis," aspiration, choking, and regurgitation of undigested food.

Diagnosis: Barium swallow (diagnostic choice) "outpouching" and upper endoscopy.

Treatment: Surgical excision (if symptomatic).

Note: NG-tubes can cause perforation in patients with esophageal diverticula.

Achalasia

Most common esophageal motility disorder. Impaired relaxation of the lower esophageal sphincter (Auerbach's/myenteric plexus [loss of inhibitory neurons]). Commonly idiopathic; occasionally caused by Chagas disease, lymphoma, or gastric carcinoma.

Hx/PE: Difficulty swallowing both solids and liquids. Chest pain and regurgitation of undigested food. Sensation of food stuck in the throat and difficulty belching (trapped air because of obstruction).

Diagnosis:

- Initial test: barium swallow ("bird beak" appearance).
- Diagnostic and most accurate test: manometry (decreased peristalsis and increased resting lower esophageal sphincter [LES] pressure).
- Endoscopy (rule out mechanical obstructions caused by malignancies).

Treatment:

- Non-specific calcium-channel blockers (first line), botulinum toxin (second line), and nitrates.
- Pneumatic balloon dilation (after medication fails), effective in 80–90% of the cases. Keep in mind the risk of perforation.
- **Heller surgery** (definitive treatment).

Gastroesophageal reflux disease (GERD)

GERD is the most common cause of chest pain. Associated with reflux of gastric content secondary to transient LES relaxation. Also associated with hiatal hernia, Barrett's esophagus, and adenocarcinoma. Metastatic conversion of the tissue from squamous to columnar cells.

Hx/PE: Heartburn 30–90 minutes after meals, which worsens with reclining and improves with anti-acids, sitting, or standing. Burning postprandial pain exacerbated by emotional stress. Dry cough in the morning with hoarseness of voice (esophagitis). No pain on palpation of the epigastric area (unlike in pancreatitis).

Diagnosis:

- Clinical diagnosis; however, if treatment fails, work-up is required.

- Most specific test: 24-hour pH monitoring (helps confirm diagnosis, if doubt).
- Upper endoscopy with biopsy in cases of unresponsiveness to treatment (might consider switching between medications first), severe pain, elderly individuals (>55 years), chronic conditions, dysphagia, odynophagia, weight loss, or GI bleeding.
- Other considerations:
  - Barium swallow (rule out hiatal hernia).
  - Esophageal manometry (rule out achalasia).

Treatment:

- First-line intervention: lifestyle modifications such as weight loss, small meals, avoiding meals three hours before bedtime, spicy foods, fatty foods, avoiding alcohol consumption, smoking, peppermint, chocolate, and some medication use. Antacids and head-of-bed elevation maybe helpful.
- First line medication: proton-pump inhibitors (inhibition of H+/K+ pump). Usually conduct a 2 months trial and re-access.
- H2-receptor antagonist (not first-line medication).
- **Nissen fundoplication** (definitive treatment); indicated when the lower esophagus is damaged or when symptoms persist despite medical therapy.

Note:

✓ PPIs needs to be given with plenty of water to decrease the side effects of nephrolithiasis.

✓ PPIs can also cause decreased absorption of calcium, increasing risk of osteoporosis.

✓ Keep in mind that therapy with H2-receptor blockers is the first-line medication for children.

Esophageal cancer

Biopsy may show formation of columnar tissue replacing native normal squamous cell tissue. Etiology and types of cancers: GERD (adenoma), Barrett's esophagus (adenoma), smoking (squamous cell), alcohol (squamous cell), and EBV (squamous cell).

➢ Upper 1/3-squamous cell (common worldwide).
➢ Lower 1/3-adenoma (common in the USA).

Hx/PE: Progressive dysphagia first with solids and then liquids, weight loss, and upper GI bleeding.

Diagnosis:

- Barium swallow (narrowing/irregular borders).
- Most accurate study: endoscopy with biopsy.
- Neck CT scan (for staging), if abnormal biopsy.

Treatment: Depends on staging; in later stages, surgical resection followed by chemotherapy (5-FU) and radiation therapy.

Barrett's esophagus

Metaplasia (reversible) of the esophageal squamous cells to intestinal-type columnar epithelium. Precursor of adenocarcinoma. Check for chronic GERD and presentation of weight loss.

Diagnosis:

- Barium swallow and upper endoscopy with biopsy (most accurate test):
  - Metaplasia (reversible), endoscopy recommended every 3–5 years.
  - Low-grade dysplasia, endoscopy recommended every 6-12 months.
  - High-grade dysphagia, ablative removal or distal esophagectomy.
- Need to rule out metastasis with chest radiography and neck/chest/abdominal CT scan.

Treatment:

- PPIs help slow progression.
- High-grade dysplasia: surgically resected and radiation and/or chemotherapy depends on staging.
- Stage III and IV (metastasis): esophageal stents and conservative management are required.

Upper GI hernias

Hiatal hernias

Diaphragmatic opening into the chest cavity, where part of the stomach pushes up into the chest cavity. Can be associated with acid reflux.

Types:

➤ Sliding hiatal hernias: gastroesophageal junction ABOVE the diaphragm.

>   Hx/PE: Sliding hernias can be associated with or without GERD.

>   Diagnosis: Chest radiography, barium swallow, or EGD.

>   Treatment: Observation, lifestyle modifications, and PPIs. Surgery unlikely, since sliding hiatal hernias are not likely to incarcerate.

➤ Paraesophageal hiatal hernias: gastroesophageal junction remains BELOW the diaphragm. These hernias are associated with a high risk of incarceration.

>   Diagnosis: Chest radiography, barium swallow, or EGD.

>   Treatment: **Surgical gastropexy** or Nissen fundoplication (decreases risk of incarceration), which prevents stomach from moving up into the chest.

Esophageal varices (dilated veins)

➤ Varices in the mid-esophagus are usually caused by compression of the superior vena cava. Patients can present with edema in the upper extremities, chest, and face.

➤ Varices in the distal esophagus are caused by hepatic cirrhosis, thrombosis of the hepatic vein, or portal hypertension.

Diagnosis:

- Upper endoscopy is diagnostic.
- Order: serial CBCs, PT/INR, PTT, platelet count, bleeding time, and type and screen.

Treatment:

- First steps are airway stabilization, IV access, and IV fluids.
- Primary prophylaxis includes non-selective β-antagonist such as propranolol (decreases blood flow and mortality) or octreotide.
- If prophylaxis medication fails, endoscopic sclerotherapy is provided (which is better than band ligation).
  - Need to give prophylactic antibiotic before endoscopy, such as IV ciprofloxacin.
- If second attempt of sclerotherapy or band ligation fails; consider correction with **transjugular intrahepatic portosystemic shunt** (TIPS).
- Hospitalized patients should be treated prophylactically with fluoroquinolones (increased risk of pneumonia, SBP, and aspiration pneumonia).

Mallory-Weiss (dilated arteries)

Sudden mucosal tear causing painless upper GI bleeding in the lower esophagus, commonly secondary to forceful retching, alcohol abuse, and a high percentage of the cases have an underling hiatal hernia.

Hx/PE: Vomiting up bright red blood, retching, and melena.

Diagnosis:

- Upper endoscopy (highly sensitive; localization of lesions).
- Order: serial CBC, PTT, PT/INR, platelet count, bleeding time, and type and screening.

Treatment:

- Usually resolves spontaneously, within 24-48 hours.
- No active bleeding, observation and supportive care is sufficient (IV fluids).
- Severe bleeding, give epinephrine injections or cauterization.
- May need blood transfusion (type and screen).

Esophageal perforation

Medical emergency

A rupture in the esophageal wall caused by trauma, infection, inflammation, endoscopy, surgery, or esophageal pathology.

Hx/PE: Acute onset of excruciating retrosternal chest pain, odynophagia (pain while swallowing), and positive Hamman's sign (crunching sound heard on palpation of the thorax due to "subcutaneous emphysema".

- Boerhaave syndrome: common in individuals with chronic alcohol consumption, with <u>full</u> thickness tear (usually lower esophagus) secondary to extreme retching and vomiting. Can present with air in subcutaneous tissue and severe pain.

Diagnosis: First, perform plain chest radiography and **gastrograffin contrast esophagram**.

Treatment:

- Prophylactic antibiotics (fluoroquinolones), IV fluids, and PPIs.
- Surgical exploration with debridement of mediastinum; closure of the perforation is an emergency.

Infectious esophagitis

➤ Candida albicans (oral thrush).

    Diagnosis:

- Physical examination: yellow/white plaques that are easy to wipe off.
- KOH: yeast/budding hyphae are diagnostic.

    Treatment: Nystatin swish and swallow or oral fluconazole.

    Note: Rule out leukoplakia (squamous cell carcinoma), DM, and HIV, unless there is an obvious cause.

➤ **Herpes simplex virus** (multiple deep painful oral ulcerations).

Diagnosis: Usually diagnosed clinically or with Tzanck test (multi-nucleated giant cells).

Treatment: Oral or topical acyclovir, not usually required.

➤ **Cytomegalovirus** (associated with esophagitis, retinitis, and colitis).

Diagnosis: Mono spot test (negative) and CMV DNA serum PCR test (specific).

Treatment: Usually resolves within 4 to 6 weeks. Mild cases might not need antiviral medication especially young and otherwise healthy patients. If the condition worsens or in case of immunosuppression, use ganciclovir.

Stomach

Gastritis

An inflammation of the stomach lining which can lead to abdominal pain, acid reflux, nausea, vomiting, and bloating.

➤ **Acute gastritis:** associated with NSAIDs, alcohol consumption, infection with *H. pylori,* and stress (burns and CNS injury).

➤ **Chronic gastritis:**

➤ **Type A chronic gastritis** (**atrophic gastritis**): autoantibodies to parietal cells (decreasing HCL and intrinsic factor). Risks of pernicious anemia and GI cancer.

➤ **Type B chronic gastritis** (90%): common in the antrum and associated with *H. pylori* infection and NSAID use.

Hx/PE: Epigastric pain usually occurring 30 minutes after a meal (patients usually experience weight loss) not relieved by anti-acids. May present with acid reflux, bloating, hematemesis, melena, and vomiting.

Diagnosis:

▪ Suspicion of *H. pylori*: urea breath test or *H. pylori* stool antigen (not routinely used).

- Suspicion of pernicious anemia: test for **anti-parietal cell antibodies** and **anti-intrinsic factor antibodies.**
- All patients with gastritis above the age of 45 years will need upper endoscopy.
- Most accurate test: upper endoscopy with biopsy.
  - Once treatment is completed, always follow-up with a second upper endoscopy to ensure the lesion has regressed.
- PPI prophylaxis for head trauma, intubation, mechanical ventilation, and burns.

Note: Pernicious anemia causes vitamin B12 deficiency.

Treatment:

- *H. pylori*-induced gastritis, use amoxicillin, clarithromycin, and omeprazole for 2 weeks.
  - If symptoms persist <u>after</u> treatment, switch antibiotic regiment to metronidazole, tetracycline, bismuth, and omeprazole.
  - If still not effective, check gastrin levels.
- Once treatment is completed, always re-scope to ensure the lesions have regressed (to rule out cancer).

Note:

✓ Female patients on misoprostol for NSAID-induced gastritis, the patient would need to use an effective method of contraception (misoprostol causes abortion).

✓ If *H. pylori* infection is associated with gastritis or ulcer disease, treat with antibiotics.

✓ If *H. pylori* infection is not the cause of ulcers or gastritis, treat underling cause and symptomatically with PPIs.

Gastric cancer

Prevalence more commonly in Asian countries. Can be caused by smoked foods, pickled foods, smoking, chronic gastritis, and *H. pylori* infection.

➤ Intestinal type: intestinal metaplasia of the gastric mucosal cells usually caused by high intake of nitrates, salts, low intake of vegetables, and *H. pylori* infection.

> **Diffuse type:** not associated with *H. pylori* infection or chronic gastritis.

Hx/PE: Epigastric pain, weight loss, melena, hematemesis, and vomiting.

Diagnosis:

- Laboratory tests include stool guaiac, stool *H. pylori* antigen, gastrin levels, and anti-parietal cell antibody.

- Upper endoscopy with biopsy (if positive biopsy findings), then perform chest, abdominal, and pelvic CT scan to determine staging.

Treatment: Depends on staging, could involve surgical excision, radiation, and chemotherapy.

Note: Video pill endoscopy is <u>inferior</u> to endoscopy for overall evaluation.

Zollinger-Ellison syndrome

Gastrin-producing tumors in the pancreas, which activates the parietal cells to release acidic secretions into the stomach. Associated with multiple ulcers in the stomach, duodenum, and jejunum. Associated with MEN I syndrome.

Hx/PE: Usually highly suspected when ulcers are <u>not</u> responsive to conventional treatments. Patients present with burning abdominal pain, diarrhea, and GI bleeding.

Diagnosis:

- Best initial test: <u>fasting</u> gastrin levels (>1000 pg/mL is diagnostic).

- If gastrin levels are not diagnostic, conduct **secretin stimulation test** (most accurate test).

  - This test, in normal circumstances, should decrease gastrin production.

- Abdominal ultrasound and abdominal CT scan.

- Highly associated with MEN I syndrome, rule out pituitary tumor and parathyroid tumor.

Treatment: High dose PPIs and surgical resection for local disease.

Small intestines

Peptic ulcer disease (PUD)

Damage to the gastric or duodenal mucosa. Most commonly caused by *H. pylori* infection, NSAIDs (second most common factor), increased gastric acid secretion, alcohol, and tobacco use. High risk of developing gastric outlet obstruction or perforation.

Hx/PE: Dull burning epigastric pain worsens 2–3 hours after a meal and pain improves with food (weight gain). "**Coffee-ground**" emesis, anemia, or hematochezia. In cases of ruptured peptic ulcers, the patient presents with peritoneal irritation, sharp constant abdominal pain, and decreased bowel sounds.

Diagnosis:

- Order: Serial CBC (if low H/H, rule out hemorrhage).
- Urea breath test, *H. pylori* stool antigen, and rectal guaiac (to rule out bleeding).
- Abdominal radiography with free air under the diaphragm (represents perforation).
  - Abdominal CT scan is the most accurate test for perforation.
- In case of gastric pain and age above 45 years, perform upper endoscopy with biopsy (to rule out cancer).

Note:

- ✓ If recurrent pain and suspected recurrent PUD; treat it as such, even if urea breath test results are negative.
- ✓ After treatment, test for *H. pylori* stool antigen (4 weeks after) or perform a urea breath test.
- ✓ Do not perform *H. pylori* serology, as this can show positive results for a year.

Treatment:

- If *H. pylori* infection: give amoxicillin, clarithromycin, and omeprazole.
- If does <u>not</u> resolve, then retest for *H. pylori*, and if results are positive, start a different regimen of antibiotics: Metronidazole,

tetracycline, bismuth, and omeprazole.

- If the patient is allergic to penicillin: use PPIs, metronidazole, and clarithromycin for 2 weeks.

- If does not resolve by conventional medications, consider pernicious anemia.

<u>In case of perforation</u>: NPO, NG-tube, IV fluids, broad-spectrum antibiotics, and emergent surgical repair. Be aware of **dumping syndrome** after surgery.

<u>Prevention</u>: All ICU, burn patients, head trauma, and intubated patients; must be given PPIs or anti-histamines to prevent stress ulcers.

Infectious diarrhea

Diarrhea

>200 g of feces with increased frequency, decreased consistency, increased motility, increased secretion, decreased osmolality, and GI inflammation.

➤ <u>Acute diarrhea:</u> lasts for <2 weeks; usually infectious (gastroenteritis) and self-limiting.

- In children, suspect rotavirus. In adults, suspect norovirus.

➤ <u>Chronic diarrhea:</u> lasts for >4 weeks; usually pathological.

- Causes: IBD, IBS, hyperthyroidism, lactose intolerance, and pancreatic insufficiency.

<u>Rule of thumb for gastric pain</u>:

➤ Infectious: "**gradual pain**," constant pain, and fever.

➤ Obstructive: "**colicky pain**," recurrent pain, increased bowel sounds, and pain improves with movement.

➤ Perforation: sudden, "**constant sharp pain**," present pain with guarding, rebound, increased pain with movement, and decreased bowel sounds.

Diagnosis:

- <u>Acute diarrhea</u>: laboratory investigation required only in case of high fever, bloody diarrhea, or if disease lasts for >4 days.

- Best initial test: fecal leukocytes and stool culture (most accurate).
- Chronic diarrhea: wide range of pathology options.
- Bloody diarrhea: may require colonoscopy.

Treatment:

- Acute diarrhea:
  - Viral pathogen: oral rehydration, loperamide (mu receptors), and bismuth salicylate.
    - ➤ Norovirus: most common virus causing infection, in adults.
  - Bacterial pathogen: antibiotics and rehydration. If infection is severe, do not wait for cultures. Consider antibiotics except in cases of *Escherichia coli* O157:H7.

Types:

➤ *Giardia lamblia*: patients with history of camping (fresh mountain streams) or also acquired by homosexual activity in men.

Prevention: boiling water before drinking.

Diagnosis: Ova or parasite culture.

Treatment: Metronidazole or if asymptomatic, no treatment required.

➤ *Staphylococcus aureus*: common history of barbecues, picnics, and potato salads. Look for combination of vomiting and diarrhea.

Treatment: usually resolves spontaneously.

➤ *Vibrio parahaemolyticus* (iron consuming): found in seafood.

Treatment: third-generation cephalosporin plus a tetracycline.

➤ *Campylobacter*: one of the most common causes of diarrhea in the United States.

Treatment: Azithromycin or tetracycline.

➤ *Salmonellosis enteritidis:* found in eggs, poultry, and meats.

Treatment: Hydration and self-limiting. Give antibiotics, if less than 1 year of age or immunosuppressed adults.

➤ *Bacillus cereus*: history of reheated fried rice, Chinese restaurants, and vomiting is common.

Treatment: Usually resolves spontaneously.

➤ *Clostridium perfringens*: reheated meat or meat that has not been refrigerated.

➤ *Cryptosporidium*: HIV patients susceptible to infection (low CD4 count). Watery diarrhea. Partially acid fast.

Treatment: HARRT medication and hydration.

➤ **Whipple disease**: diarrhea, malabsorption, and weight loss.

Diagnosis: Most accurate test: Bowel biopsy (PAS-positive organism).

Treatment: TMP-SMX is curative.

➤ Amebic: parasite invasion can cause liver abscess.

Treatment: Metronidazole.

➤ Chronic diarrhea: identify underlying cause and treat accordingly.

Note:

✓ Diet for diarrhea needs to be age appropriate with low intake of simple sugars and low fat.

✓ Metronidazole is the best medication for GI anaerobes, and clindamycin is the best medication for respiratory anaerobes.

✓ Probiotics taken with antibiotic treatment can help decrease the risk of diarrhea.

Infectious diarrhea pathogens

*Work-up and antibiotic treatment are not usually needed for infectious diarrhea. Work-up needed in cases of moderate to severe symptoms, bloody diarrhea, high fever, or diarrhea lasting longer than 4 days.

➤ *Campylobacter*

Usually causes acute diarrhea in young adults and might present with bloody diarrhea. Infection can be transferred via fecal-oral route, contaminated water, or food products.

Diagnosis: Stool culture (elevated RBCs and WBCs). Keep in mind that stool cultures can take a few days.

Treatment:

- Self-limiting or oral azithromycin (if severe disease or immunosuppressed status).
- Common measures are to increase fluid intake, maintain good hygiene, and decrease fats and sugars in the diet (as these can exacerbate diarrhea).

Note: In case of nausea and vomiting, give anti-emetics.

➤ *Clostridium difficile*

Watery smelly diarrhea can occur about 2 weeks after antibiotic treatment with clindamycin (most common), cephalosporins, fluoroquinolones, or penicillin.

Hx/PE: Presents with abdominal pain, steatorrhea, low-grade fever, and watery diarrhea.

Diagnosis:

- PCR or ELISA stool culture for *C. difficile* antigen.
- In cases of negative test results, perform sigmoidoscopy (may show **pseudomembranous**). Study can be of use when diagnoses is uncertain or does not improve with standard treatment.

Treatment:

- Oral metronidazole (typically first line) or oral vancomycin (alternative).

- Treat first episode with oral metronidazole (cost effective) three times a day for 10 days.
- If unresolved after treatment with metronidazole, then use oral vancomycin.
- In case of toxicity or creatinine level >1.5 from the baseline or leukocytosis >15,000/µL, then administer oral vancomycin.
- **Pregnant women** with *C. difficile* infection, use oral vancomycin.
- Indicate preventive measures such as hand washing with soap and water.

➤ *Entamoeba histolytica* (ameba)

An anaerobic parasitic protozoan that can cause hepatic abscess. More common in men with a history of recent travel to developing countries.

Hx/PE: Patients present with fever and RUQ abdominal pain.

Diagnosis:
- First test: RUQ abdominal ultrasonography (liver abscess).
- CBC (elevated leukocytes), alkaline phosphatase, and liver enzymes (can be normal).
- Serum entamoeba histolytica antibody test (sensitive in 95% of the cases).
- Stool culture (less sensitive) and only diagnostic in about 15% of the cases.

Treatment: Oral metronidazole three times a day for 10 days. If the condition does not resolve, surgical drainage is needed (rarely done).

Note: Do not give steroids to patients with *Entamoeba histolytica*, as steroids can cause perforation.

➤ *Escherichia coli O157:H7*

Linked to raw contaminated vegetables, undercooked meat, and unpasteurized milk. Can be associated with HUS, especially in younger and elderly patients. If patients develop

HUS, they may require blood transfusion (hemoglobin < 6 g/dL).

Diagnosis: Stool culture (not routinely used).

Treatment: Supportive care only (hydration and electrolytes). Do not give anti-diarrheal or antibiotics medications. Usually self-limiting within 5-10 days.

Note: Never give antibiotics or anti-diarrheal therapy (loperamide) to patients with *E. coli* 0157:H7, as these treatments can cause HUS.

➤ *Salmonella*

A gram-negative bacteria found in poultry products, pork, and eggs. Salmonella can hide in the liver and can cause osteomyelitis in sickle-cell disease patients. Can be associated with gallbladder cancer.

Hx/PE: Abdominal pain, possible bloody diarrhea, and dehydration.

Diagnosis: Stool culture and stool guaiac.

Treatment:

- Supportive therapy (fluids) and good hygiene (hand washing).
- In case of severe disease, high fever, or immunosuppressed status, give oral TMP-SMX or quinolones.
- Avoid anti-diarrheal therapy, as these medications can worsen course.

➤ *Shigella*

Gram-negative facultative anaerobic bacteria that can be transmitted via fecal-oral route from human host.

Hx/PE: Bloody diarrhea and severe dehydration.

Diagnosis: Stool culture and stool guaiac.

Treatment:

- Supportive therapy (fluids) and good hygiene (hand washing).

- In case of severe disease, high fever, or immunosuppressed status, give oral TMP-SMX or quinolones.
- Avoid anti-diarrheal therapy, as these medications can worsen course.

➤ *Yersinia enterocolitica*

Gram-negative bacteria transmitted via fecal-oral route and primarily located in the terminal ileum. Rule out appendicitis, if high suspicion.

Hx/PE: Watery diarrhea and RLQ pain (resembling appendicitis).

Diagnosis: CBC (leukocytosis) and stool culture.

Treatment: Self-limiting and does not usually require treatment. If sever infection consider TMP-SMX or fluoroquinolones.

➤ *Echinococcus*

A parasitic disease transmitted by a parasite. Common vectors are dogs which causes "hydatid cysts" in humans.

Diagnosis: RUQ abdominal ultrasonography, abdominal CT scan (eggshell calcification), and stool culture.

Treatment: Surgical removal of cysts and albendazole and/or mebendazole (before and after surgery).

➤ Roundworm, pinworms, and hookworms

Parasitic infections that can develop into megaloblastic anemia and malabsorption (diarrhea).

Diagnosis: CBC (eosinophilia), electrolytes, stool culture (parasites), and MCV testing (>100 um^3).

Treatment: Albendazole or mebendazole.

Malabsorption

Malabsorption

Inability to absorb nutrients. Can be attributed to many pathologies such as chronic pancreatitis, Whipple disease, and celiac sprue.

Hx/PE: Frequent bowel movements, loose watery stools, foul smelling bulky stools, flatus, and bloating.

Diagnosis:

- CBC, electrolytes, and stool culture (fat, osmolality, and pH). Malabsorption can be attributed to many pathologies, be selective in your clinical diagnostic tools.
- Best initial test is **Sudan black stain** of stool (measures fat).
- Most sensitive test is 72-hour fecal fat test.

Treatment:

- Etiology dependent and a confirmed diagnosis is required before preparing treatment plan.
- Consider nutrients via TPN, PEG tube, or central line.

Note: Enteral feeding→ Standard composition is 30 kcal·kg^{-1}·day^{-1} and 1 g·kg^{-1}·day^{-1} of protein.

Lactose intolerance

Lactose intolerance is due to a decrease in the level of lactase, a brush-boarder enzyme. Lactose sugars are converted to glucose + galactose by the enzyme lactase. Common in Africans, Asians, and Native Americans.

Hx/PE: Abdominal bloating, flatulence, cramping, and watery diarrhea after milk ingestion, all of which resolve in 24 hours.

Diagnosis: **Hydrogen breath test** (elevated), stool osmolality (elevated), and stool pH (low). Diarrhea will subside within 24–48 hours after stopping lactose.

Treatment:

- Avoid dairy products or give lactase enzyme replacement.

- If intake of dairy products are reduced consider calcium and vitamin D supplementation, as milk products contain added high levels of calcium.
- Yogurt does not contain high levels of lactose.

Note: Before taking a hydrogen breath test, the patient needs to be fasting for at least 8 hours.

Carcinoid syndrome

Hormone-producing enterochromaffin cells. Increased metabolism of tryptophan to serotonin. Serotonin is metabolized (degraded) to 5-hydroxyindoleacetic acid (5-HIAA).

Hx/PE: Symptoms usually occur after eating or strong emotion and presents with cutaneous flushing (most commonly), diarrhea, bronchoconstriction (wheezing), and heart failure (right-sided cardiac valves).

Diagnosis: Most useful test: 24-hour urine levels of serotonin (5-HIAA). Octreotide scan used to localize tumor.

Treatment:
- Octreotide (somatostatin analog) slows tumor growth and inhibits serotonin secretion by the tumor.
- Surgical resection of the tumor and chemotherapy.

Note: Octreotide also inhibits growth hormone, gastrin, insulin, and glucagon. Is used to treat insulinoma, glucagonoma, acromegalia, carcinoid tumor, and esophageal varices.

Irritable bowel syndrome (IBS)

Irritable bowel syndrome

An idiopathic functional disorder of the gut-brain axis and over growth of bacteria in the small intestines. Symptoms worsen with stress and can be associated with psychiatric disorders. IBS can be triggered by acute gastroenteritis infection.

Hx/PE: <u>Alternating</u> diarrhea and constipation with mild abdominal pain that is relieved by bowel movements.

Diagnosis: Diagnosis of exclusion: CBC, electrolytes, TSH, abdominal ultrasound, stool culture, and colonoscopy. Laboratory evaluation which normal results.

Treatment:

- Increase fluids, fiber intake, probiotics, and SSRIs.
- Diarrhea: anti-diarrheal medication (loperamide).
- Constipation: docusate or antispasmodics (anticholinergics).

Note: Loperamide is also known as Imodium.

Bowel obstructions

Small bowel obstruction

Complete or partial obstruction of the colon can lead to ischemia or necrosis of the bowel. Patients commonly present with hyperactive bowel sounds, distended proximal bowel loops, electrolyte imbalance, and fluid disruption.

Risk factors: adhesions (60%), hernia (15%), neoplasm, constipation, volvulus, intussusception, IBD, CF, and strictures.

➤ **Partial bowel obstruction** (flatus with no stool passage).

➤ **Complete bowel obstruction** (no flatus and no stool passage).

Hx/PE: Abdominal pain described as "colicky," which tend to improve with movement. Can present with emesis, fever, dehydration, hypotension, peristaltic waves, and "high-pitched" bowel sounds.

Diagnosis:

- CBC, electrolytes, lactic acid (elevated if bowel necrosis), BUN/ Cr ratio (elevated if dehydrated), abdominal radiography (rule out perforations), gastrografin contrast study, and abdominal CT scan.
- If surgery required order, platelets, PT/INR, PTT, bleeding time, and type and cross.

Note: Gastrografin contrast study, is water soluble.

Treatment:

- Partial obstruction: admit for observation and stabization. Place NG-tube, NPO, IV fluids, analgesics, antiemetics, correct electrolytes, and Foley catheter placement (measure ins and outs). If fails to improve within 12-24 hours consider surgical intervention.

- Complete or necrotic obstruction: **emergency surgery** and prophylaxis antibiotics.

- In case of peritoneal signs or guarding, go straight to surgery (laparoscopy).

Large bowel obstruction

Can be partial or complete obstruction of the colon. This pathology is caused by physical obstruction, whereas ileus is not a physical obstruction.

Risk factors: adhesions, diverticulitis, tumors, volvulus, intussusception, and fecal impaction.

Hx/PE: Proximal distention, tenderness, "high-pitched" bowel sounds. Rule out peritoneal sign (perforations).

Diagnosis:

- CBC, electrolytes, BUN/Cr ratio (elevated if dehydrated), and lactic acid level testing (elevated in case of bowel ischemia).

- Abdominal radiography (rule out perforations) and abdominal CT scan (diagnostic).

- If stable, can consider colonoscopy, depending on the pathology.

- If surgery required order, PT/INR, PTT, bleeding time, platelets, and type and cross.

Treatment:

- If stable, hospitalize, give gastric rest (NPO), NG-tube, IV fluids, analgesics, antiemetic's, and place Foley catheter.

- In case of peritoneal signs (rebound or guarding), go straight to **emergency surgery** and prophylaxis antibiotics.

- If secondary to fecal impaction, give enemas and suppositories followed by fiber and fluid intake.

Ileus

Decreased <u>or</u> no bowel sounds or bowel movements and "**no structural obstruction**."

<u>Risk factors</u>: Recent GI surgery, GI procedure, immobility, hypokalemia, electrolyte imbalance, hypothyroidism, diabetes, and medication.

Hx/PE: <u>Absence</u> of flatulence or bowel movements, positive abdominal distention, and no peritoneal signs. Ileus symptoms are different from those of small and large bowel obstruction. With ileus there are decreased or no bowel sounds and no structural obstruction.

Diagnosis:
- CBC, electrolytes, lactic acid, TSH, HbA1c, and abdominal radiography (distended loops of small or large bowel, with no obstruction).
- Gastrografin study (to rule out obstruction).
- **Gastric emptying study** (decreased bowel movements).

Note: With ileus rule out diabetes (fasting glucose levels), hypothyroidism (TSH and FT4), medications, and electrolyte abnormalities.

Treatment:
- NPO, NG-tube, correct electrolytes, and TPN.
- Erythromycin, lactulose, and neostigmine help increase bowel movements.
- Discontinue narcotics (mu receptor narcotics) <u>or</u> other medications causing ileus.
- Treat underlying diabetes or thyroid dysfunction.

Ogilvie syndrome

A type of pseudo-obstruction seen in elderly patients who are immobile or post-operative. Can have electrolyte abnormalities (low K+, Mg+2, or Ca+2). Need to rule out cancer and other causes.

: Abdominal pain, decrease bowel sounds, abdominal distention, nausea, and constipation.

Diagnosis:

- CBC, electrolytes, TSH, HgA1c, abdominal radiography (dilated megacolon), and gastrografin study (which is different from barium study, as gastrografin study iswater soluble and less corrosive).
- Gastric emptying study (decreased bowel movements).
- Rule out diabetes (HbA1c), hypothyroidism (TSH and FT4), and review medications.

Treatment: Correct electrolyte abnormalities and use prokinetic agents (administer IV neostigmine).

Note: Neostigmine can cause bradycardia and bronchospasms, which can be reversed by atropine.

Dumping syndrome

Abnormally rapid release of gastric content (undigested content) into the duodenum.

Risk factors: patients with previous GI surgery.

Hx/PE: Nausea, vomiting, diarrhea, and lightheadedness.

Diagnosis:

- A clinical diagnosis more commonly with a history of gastrectomy.
- Gastrografin study and gastric emptying study.

Treatment:

- High-protein, low-carbohydrate (simple sugars), and small frequent meals.
- Fluids should be taken between meals, not during meals. Fluids during meals can accelerate gastric emptying.

Bowel ischemia

Mesenteric ischemia

Most common site of obstruction is the superior mesenteric artery (secondary to location and angle). Obstruction decreases the mesenteric blood supply (intestinal angina) causing ischemic injury and acute or chronic arterial occlusion. Look for risk factors of coagulopathy.

Risk factors: atrial fibrillation, cardiac hypokinesis, and hypercoagulable states.

Hx/PE: Sever sudden abdominal pain "out of proportion" to palpation on physical exam. Look for peritoneal signs, cramping lower abdominal pain, nausea, vomiting, and bloody stool.

Diagnosis:

- CBC, electrolytes, lactic acid (rule out metabolic acidosis), LDH, blood culture (rule out sepsis), and CPK.
- Abdominal radiography and abdominal CT scan, "thumb printing," bowel edema, and pneumatosis intestinalis.
- Most accurate test: **mesenteric angiography.**
- May need colonoscopy with biopsy, but the pathology report takes time.

Note: Early mesenteric angiogram is the most appropriate diagnostic step but exploratory laparotomy is the preferred choice when an angiogram cannot be performed or when the condition has progressed and the patient has acidosis secondary to necrosis.

Treatment:

- NPO, NG-tube, IV fluids, and broad-spectrum antibiotics.
- Treatment options: anti-coagulation medication, angioplasty, thrombectomy, or endovascular stenting.
    - If diagnosed during surgery, use embolectomy.
    - If diagnosed during angiography, use thrombolytics (if no contraindications).
- Deterioration or peritoneal signs: Laparotomy and resection of necrotic bowel.
- Keep in mind that IV fluids and antibiotics are the first step.

Large bowel pathologies

Diverticulosis

A false diverticula (outpouching of only the mucosa and submucosa) and is the most common cause of massive lower GI bleeding in elderly patients. Associated with low-fiber diet, high-fat diet, and constipation.

Risk factors: older age individuals with low fluid intake, low-fiber diet, and high-fat diet. Can be a complication of a single diverticular arteriole (erosion of the artery).

Hx/PE: Sudden "painless bright red GI bleeding."

Diagnosis:

- CBC (serial), electrolytes, stool guaiac test, colonoscopy, abdominal CT scan, and barium enema (more accurate test than colonoscopy).
- PTT, PT/INR, bleeding time, platelets, and cross and type.
- Blood transfusion could be the first step to treat symptomatic patients.

Note: All patients scheduled for a colonoscopy need to be NPO and given IV fluids.

Treatment:

- If hospitalized: gastric rest (NPO), NG-tube, IV fluids, and transfusions (PRBC), as needed.
- In elderly patients with symptomatic anemia, consider transfusion (to keep hemoglobin above 10) before procedures or standard treatments.
- Outpatient diet: high-fiber, low fat diet, and high fluid intake (if no contraindications).
- Angiogram required, if bleeding continues and surgical consideration.

Diverticulitis

Inflammation of diverticula in the lower GI tract, with the potential to cause abscess or perforation. If a young female presents with lower abdominal pain, need to consider ectopic pregnancy and ovarian torsion.

Risk factors: common in elderly patients who have a low-fiber, high-fat diet, and low water intake.

Hx/PE: "Painful with no GI bleeding," gradual onset of left lower quadrant abdominal pain and fever. In cases of sigmoid diverticulitis, abscess formation is the most common complication.

Diagnosis:

- CBC: leukocytosis (inflammation) and H/H (rule out bleeding).
- Abdominal radiography: rule out perforation, ileus, or obstruction.
- The best and most accurate test is abdominal CT scan.
- If no improvement, rule out abscess or perforation.
- Colonoscopy or barium enema are contraindicated in diverticulitis because of high risk of perforation.

Note:

✓ Preparation for CT scan: discontinue NSAIDs, check renal function (BUN/Cr ratio), and give normal saline hydration before contrast.

✓ In cases of heart failure, caution with the amount of fluids given.

Treatment:

- If patient is stable, treat as outpatient with oral antibiotics for 7 to 10 days and special diet.
- If patient is unstable or elderly, hospitalize and place NPO, NG-tube, IV fluids, broad-spectrum antibiotics (metronidazole and fluoroquinolones or cephalosporin), and analgesics.
- In case of perforation or abscess, surgical repair is required.

Appendicitis

Medical emergency

Fecalith obstruction of the appendiceal orifice causing inflammation. More common in younger patients. Consider ovarian torsion and ectopic pregnancy.

Hx/PE: Triad: Fever, leukocytosis, and RLQ abdominal pain. Other symptoms are nausea, vomiting, and decreased appetite.

Physical examination:

- **Rovsing's sign:** palpation of the LLQ causes pain in the RLQ.
- **Psoas sign**: RLQ pain with thigh extension.

Diagnosis:

- If high clinical diagnosis (high fever, elevated CBC, and RLQ pain): no need for abdominal CT scan.
- Most accurate test is abdominal CT scan (confirms diagnosis).
- Use ultrasound in pregnancy cases.
- Also, consider ectopic pregnancy and ovarian torsion work-up, if stable.

Treatment:

- Place patient NPO, NG-tube, IV fluids, analgesics, and IV antibiotics immediately (before appendectomy).
- <u>Atypical</u> presentation, perform abdominal CT scan first.
- High suspicion <u>or</u> typical presentation of appendicitis, go straight to emergency **laparoscopic appendectomy**, even before abdominal CT scan.

Note: Perforation of appendices can lead to septic shock.

Hemorrhoids

External hemorrhoids

Often caused by heavy lifting, constipation, or labor. Symptoms usually do not last for more than 3 days and this is the time frame for intervention with prophylactic treatment.

Hx/PE: Rectal pain, bright red rectal bleeding (rare), and nodes felt with external digital examination (more common at 6 o'clock position), and <u>no</u> change in stool caliber.

Diagnosis: Physical examination (diagnostic) or anoscopy.

Treatment:
- For symptomatic relief, patients can have warm water baths and NSAIDs.

- Little evidence on use of suppositories (hydrocortisone with lidocaine).
- If suppository steroids are used, do not use for longer than 14 days.
  - Definitive treatment with **sclerotherapy** or surgical excision.
  - Long-term prophylaxis: increase fiber intake.

Note: Sclerotherapy can be used for spider veins, varicose veins, and hemorrhoids.

Internal hemorrhoids

Hx/PE: <u>Non</u>-painful rectal bleeding during or following bowel movements and no change in stool caliber.

Diagnosis:
- <u>Stable</u>: anoscopy or sigmoidoscopy.
- <u>Unstable</u>: angiogram or laparotomy (rare).

Treatment: Definitive treatment with **rubber band ligation**.

Colon cancers

Colon and rectal cancer

- ➤ Rectal cancer is the third leading cause of cancer in <u>both</u> men and women and the third leading cause of mortality in the USA after lung cancer.
- ➤ Patients aged above 50 years with anemia and positive stool guaiac test; will need a colonoscopy to rule out colon cancer.
- ➤ If HIV positive status, consider rectal squamous cell carcinoma.
- ➤ Villous polyps are aggressive polyps. Need to rule out celiac disease, which can present with villous atrophy.
- ➤ Tubular polyps are less progressive than villous polyps.

<u>Risk factors:</u> genetic causes, ulcerative colitis, Crohn's disease, high-fat diet, low-fiber diet, diabetes, obesity, alcohol, and smoking. Usually need history of heavy and long-term alcohol and smoking abuse.

Cancer locations and presentation:

- Right side cancer: anemia, occult blood, and obstruction rare.
- Left side cancer: obstruction, decrease stool caliber, and constipation.
- Rectal lesions: bright red blood.

Colon cancer overall diagnosis:

- CBC, electrolytes, and stool guaiac test.
- Left sided lesions: sigmoidoscopy with biopsy (all positive sigmoidoscopies, will need to be followed with full colonoscopy).
- Right sided lesions: colonoscopy with biopsy (all positive colonoscopies, will need to be followed by upper endoscopy).
- PET scan: used to view the metabolic activity of malignant tumors (tumors use high levels of glucose). Measure glucose levels prior to PET scan to rule out diabetes, as it can produce false positive results).
- Metastatic work-up: chest/abdominal/pelvic CT scan, chest radiography, alkaline phosphates, and LFTs.

Colon cancer overall treatment:

- Surgical resection, regional lymph node dissection (staging purposes), radiation therapy (not routinely used for colon cancer), and chemotherapy (if positive lymph nodes).
- Follow up with CEA levels for monitoring recurrence (measure every 3-6 months for the first 2 years after surgery; and then every 6 month for the next 5 years). Also follow-up with pelvic, abdominal, and chest CT scan, annually for the first 3 years.

Note: Patients will have a risk of adhesions after GI surgery.

➤ **Peutz-Jeghers syndrome**

Autosomal dominate (AD), benign, non-malignant hamartomatous polyps in the small and large intestines. Skin hyperpigmentation on the hands, perioral region, and buccal mucosa.

Treatment: Resection of the polyps is required only if serious bleeding.

➤ Familial adenomatous polyposis (FAP)

AD, mutation of *APC gene,* hundreds to thousands of polyps with inevitable (100%) colorectal cancer by the age of 45 years.

Diagnosis:

- Patients with a family history need to undergo genetic testing (*APC gene*) and yearly colonoscopies. Start colonoscopy screening between the age of 10 and 12 years.
- These patients will need <u>both</u> colonoscopy and upper endoscopy.

Treatment: **Total proctocolectomy** (indicated when polyps are detected).

➤ Gardner's syndrome

AD, mutation of the *APC gene*, hundreds to thousands of colonic polyps, 100% likelihood of colon cancer before the age of 50 years. Associated with osteoma tumors and congenital hypertrophy of the retinal pigment epithelium.

Treatment: Surgery, palliative care, and chemotherapy (not very affective)

➤ Turcot syndrome

AD, mutation of the *APC gene*, associated with CNS tumors such as medulloblastoma.

➤ Hereditary nonpolyposis colorectal cancer (HNPCC) or Lynch syndrome

AD, high risk of colon cancer (80%), and affected women have a high risk of developing endometrial cancer or ovarian cancer.

Treatment: First line treatment is surgery.

➤ MALT lymphoma

Secondary to *H. pylori* infection; typically has a good prognosis and infrequently progresses to a diffuse large B-cell lymphoma.

Treatment: Amoxicillin, clarithromycin, and omeprazole. In rare cases radiation and chemotherapy.

➤ **Gastric adenocarcinoma with Krukenberg tumor**

A metastatic "signet ring" cell adenocarcinoma arising in the stomach and metastasizing to the ovaries (commonly bilateral).

Treatment: Removal of ovaries, radiation, and chemotherapy.

GI bleeding

Upper GI bleeding

Risk factors: esophagitis, esophageal perforation, esophageal varices, Mallory Weiss tears, gastritis, gastric ulcers, and PUD.

Hx/PE: Hematemesis, melena, chocking, coughing, and SOB.

Diagnosis:

- First steps: stabilize patient (ABCs) and assessment of vital signs.
- Serial CBCs (anemia), electrolytes, PT/INR, PTT, bleeding time, platelet count, typing and screen, and stool guaiac test.
- NPO, IV fluids, NG-tube, and NG-lavage.
- Upper endoscopy (if stable), avoid perforation.

Treatment:

- Protect airway, give IV fluids, and PRBC (as needed, highly consider if <7g/dL).
- Considerations depend on etiology and stability of patient:
  - PUD (antibiotics and PPIs), esophagitis (stop irritant), esophageal perforation (antibiotics and surgery), esophageal varices (sclerotherapy, octreotide, or propranolol), and Mallory Weiss tears (epinephrine injections).
- If patient is intubated, give PPIs to prevent stress ulceration.
- Place on respiratory precautions.

Lower GI bleeding

Considered a lower GI bleed, if occurs distal to the ligament of Treitz.

Hx/PE: Clinical presentation will vary from bright red blood to melena, which will depend on the location of the bleeding source.

Diagnosis:

- Initial steps are evaluation of stability and assessment of vital signs.
- CBC, electrolytes, stool guaiac test, PT/INR, PTT, bleeding time, and cross and type.
- First need to consider ruling out upper GI bleeding with NG-lavage.
- Check orthostatics to help monitor blood loss.
- Colonoscopy is the test of choice in most cases of acute lower GI bleeding.
- Monitor bleeding: serial CBC (anemia) and consider:
  - Bleeding >2 mL/min – perform angiogram.
  - Bleeding 0.5–2 mL/min – use tagged RBC.
  - Bleeding <0.5 mL/min or not actively bleeding – perform colonoscopy.

Treatment: Treat underlying cause.

Note: Barium enemas are contraindicated during active bleeding.

Inflammatory bowel diseases

Ulcerative colitis (UC)

A type of inflammatory bowel disease (IBD) with colon and rectal involvement. The inflammation is limited to the mucosa and submucosa. Can be exacerbated by stress and emotion.

Extraintestinal manifestations: uveitis (painful blurry vision), arthritis, primary sclerosing cholangitis (PSC), erythema nodosum (EN), p-ANCA, and colorectal cancer. About 80% of the patients with PSC have ulcerative colitis.

Hx/PE: Fever, bloody diarrhea (common), abdominal cramps, weight loss, and orthostatic hypotension.

Diagnosis:

- CBC (rule out infection), electrolyte (electrolyte abnormalities), and stool culture (infection).
- Abdominal radiography (to rule out perforations).
- Barium enema can be diagnostic.
- Colonoscopy (continuous rectal involvement, loss of the vascular appearance of the colon, and pseudopolyps).
- Most accurate test is biopsy (inflammation of crypts).
- **Toxic megacolon**: dilated transverse colon and absent or altered haustra.
- In case of high suspicion of toxic megacolon, rule out infectious causes.

Treatment:

- Best initial therapy: mesalamine.
- 5-ASA (sulfasalazine rectal): rectal preferred over oral but can consider combination.
- If no improvement is observed, budesonide (acute symptoms) is preferred over prednisone.
- Azathioprine (in case of relapse or severe disease).
- **Total proctocolectomy** (removal of the rectum and part of or the entire colon) is curative of toxic megacolon, chronic use of steroids, multiple hospitalizations, or colon cancer.
- Toxic megacolon: avoid 5-ASAs (can precipitate attacks) and give glucocorticoids.

Prevention:

- Colonoscopy screening for FAP carcinoma starts at 12 years of age, and for ulcerative colitis screening starts 8 years after diagnosis.
- Toxic megacolon: first start with conservative medical management for 24–48 hours with IV steroids, IV fluids, antibiotics, and IV cyclosporine. However, if the condition

worsens, definitive treatment is colectomy before perforated bowel develops.

Note: Mesalamine enemas (active ingredient is 5-ASA) are effective in reducing inflammation and preferred over steroid suppositories.

Crohn's disease

A type of inflammatory bowel disease (IBD) that can occur within <u>any</u> portion of the GI tract from the mouth to the anus; more commonly in the ileocecal region. Patients present with discontinuous pattern (skipping lesions), "transmural inflammation," and often rectum is spared. Patients can have oral ulcers.

<u>Extraintestinal manifestations</u>: uveitis, arthritis, erythema nodosum, PSC, gallstones, nephrolithiasis, and fistulas in the bladder or bowel loops (not observed in ulcerative colitis).

Hx/PE: Decreased absorption of water and fat-soluble vitamins (D, E, A, K). Macrocytic anemia caused by decreased vitamin B12 absorption. Abdominal pain, weight loss, watery diarrhea, and mild fever.

Diagnosis:
- CBC (rule out anemia and infection), electrolytes, stool culture (rule out infections), and stool guaiac test.
- Barium enema can be diagnostic.
- Colonoscopy (ulcers, "cobblestones," "skipping lesions," and "creeping fat").
- Biopsy (gold standard) with **non-caseating granulomas** (specific).

Treatment:
- Best initial therapy: mesalamine.
- Sulfasalazine (5-ASA) better rectal than oral.
- Medication options: corticosteroids (acute exacerbations), azathioprine (used for long-term therapy and severe cases), and infliximab.
- Antibiotics (metronidazole and ciprofloxacin) during episodes of diarrhea, abscesses, and fistulas.
- Vitamin and mineral supplementation: vitamin B12 (decreased

with Crohn's disease), calcium and vitamin D (decreased with steroid use and Crohn's disease), iron (decrease by bleeding).

- Surgical resection (for fistula, abscess, or perforation).

Note: Need to rule out tuberculosis with infliximab use.

Lower GI hernias

Inguinal hernias

High risk of incarceration and strangulation.

Hesselbach's triangle: inguinal ligament, rectus abdominals, and inferior epigastric artery.

- **Indirect hernia** (most common).
  Herniation through <u>both</u> internal and external inguinal rings, lateral to the inferior epigastric artery, and progressing to the scrotum.

- **Direct hernia (Hesselbach).**
  Herniation only through external ring and medial to the inferior epigastric artery.

Hx/PE: Suspect bowel strangulation when present with fever, leukocytosis, and lower abdominal pain.

Diagnosis:

- <u>Stable</u>: CBC, electrolytes, lactic acid, abdominal ultrasonography, and abdominal CT scan.

- <u>Unstable</u> (if fever or cannot reduce hernia): immediate surgery.

Note: Do not try to reduce hernia, if elevated leukocytes, abdominal pain, or fever.

Treatment:

- First step if unstable: IV fluids and gastric rest (NPO).

- If hernia does not resolve or fever is present, immediate surgery will be required.

- Direct hernia: correct transversalis fascia.
- Indirect hernia: reduce the size of the internal inguinal ring, so only the spermatic cord passes through it.
- Surgical management (open or laparoscopic).

Note: Femoral hernias have a higher risk of strangulation than inguinal hernias.

Fistulas

Fistula-in-ano

An opening of the cutaneous surface near the anus, which can communicate with the rectum, and presences of granular tissue. High risk of development after anal abscesses.

Hx/PE: Pain during defecation and soiling of underwear despite no defecation.

Diagnosis: Clinical diagnosis, anoscopy, or sigmoidoscopy.

Treatment: **Fistulotomy** (surgery).

Colovesical fistula

Risk factors: include diverticulitis, Crohn's disease, or trauma.

Hx/PE: "Pneumaturia" and recurrent UTIs.

Diagnosis: Urinalysis, urine culture, and abdominal/pelvic CT scan with contrast (best imaging study to start work-up).

Treatment: Antibiotics and surgery.

Gallbladder diseases

Acute cholecystitis

Cholecystits is due to "prolonged" blockage of the cystic duct by gallstones (cholelithiasis), leading to inflammation and distention of the gallbladder (cholecystitis), which causes elevated pressure and RUQ pain. Most gallstones are cholesterol stones, which are radiolucent.

In case of **acalculous cholecystitis,** there are <u>no</u> stones but only a thickened gallbladder wall. The patients are usually on TPN, experiencing septic shock, or chronically ill (burn or trauma victims).

Hx/PE: Patients are asymptomatic at first, and later present with low-grade fever, nausea, vomiting, constant pain, and mild icterus. Patients can develop gangrene gallbladder because of infection.

- Murphy's sign: RUQ pain on palpation (most accurate sign), sensitive but not specific.

- Obturator sign: internal rotation of the right thigh.

- Psoas sign: extension of the hip.

Diagnosis:

- CBC (elevated WBC count), alkaline phosphatase (usually normal), ALT and AST levels (usually normal), bilirubin levels (usually normal), and ultrasonography (thickened gallbladder with stones and/or bile sludge).

- Perform a **hepatic iminodiacetic acid level testing** (HIDA scan) also known as **cholescintigraphy** when ultrasonography findings are equivocal.

Note:

- ✓ HIDA scan and ultrasonography are better for detecting stones in the *cystic ducts.*

- ✓ Magnetic resonance cholangiopancreatography (MRCP) is better for visualizing stones in the *common bile ducts.*

Treatment:

- First steps: pain control (narcotics), IV fluids administration, and board-spectrum antibiotic administration, such as Zosyn or cephalosporins <u>plus</u> fluoroquinolones.

- Clinically <u>stable</u> patients with acute cholecystitis and no progression of fever, with normal vital signs, and no signs of perforation can undergo a cholecystectomy within 24–48 hours, if the condition is unresolved.
- If the patient is <u>unstable</u>, perform immediate cholecystectomy; give IV fluids, NPO, IV antibiotics, and perform **laparoscopic cholecystectomy**.

<u>Prevention</u>:

➤ Rapid weight loss can increase the likelihood of stone formation.

➤ Low-carbohydrate diet and increased physical activity can help prevent gallstone formation.

Note: Development of bile duct strictures are common after laparoscopic cholecystectomy.

Cholelithiasis

These are gallstones in the actual gallbladder that can spread to the cystic duct or common bile duct. These stones are associated with an increased risk of gallbladder perforation or infections.

<u>Risk factors</u>: "5 Fs": female gender, fat, forty, fertile, and flatulence. OCP use, rapid weight loss, family history, chronic hemolysis, Native American ethnicity, and TPN use.

Hx/PE: RUQ pain radiating to the right subscapular area (secondary to increase in gallbladder pressure). Patient can experience <u>intermittent</u> postprandial pain, fatty food intolerance, nausea, vomiting, and flatulence.

Diagnosis: laboratory tests: CBC (mild leukocytosis), ALT and AST levels (not elevated), alkaline phosphate level (not elevated), bilirubin levels (usually not elevated), and RUQ ultrasonography (85–90% sensitive) or HIDA scan.

Note: Ultrasonography is fast and cheap and usually the first choice.

Treatment:

- <u>Asymptomatic</u>: dietary modification with no further

interventions. **Ursodeoxycholic acid** can sometimes help dissolve small cholesterol stones.

- Symptomatic: laparoscopic cholecystectomy (curative).

Fun facts:

- After a cholecystectomy, there is no need for diet modifications other than for health reasons.

- Patient can experience transient episodes of flatulence and diarrhea. Give **cholestyramine** (bile salt-binding resin) which binds to bile salts and can help with diarrhea.

- If surgery is necessary order: PTT, PT/INR, platelet count, bleeding time, cross and type, and patient's written consent.

Choledocholithiasis

Gallstones in the *common bile duct*.

Stone types:

➤ **Cholesterol stones:** most common type of gallstones accounting for almost 80–85% of stones.

➤ **Black pigmented stones**: caused by chronic *hemolysis* (hemoglobin breaks down), including sickle-cell anemia.

➤ **Brown pigmented stones:** often caused by chronic *infection*. Composed of small amounts of proteins, cholesterol, bilirubin, and calcium salts.

Hx/PE: Biliary colic, jaundice, fever, and possible pancreatitis.

Diagnosis:

- CBC (leukocytosis), ALT and AST levels (elevated), alkaline phosphatase level (markedly elevated), total bilirubin levels (elevated), amylase and lipase level (elevation will depend on how distal the stones are), and abdominal ultrasonography or HIDA scan.

- If the HIDA scan is not diagnostic then ERCP can be performed.

Note: As a rule of thumb, stones in the *cystic duct* will usually have normal laboratory results. Stones in the *common bile duct* or further downstream will have elevated bilirubin, alkaline phosphatase, and liver enzymes.

Treatment:

- Endoscopic retrograde sphincterotomy (ERS) followed by ERCP or lithotripsy (extracorporeal shock wave lithotripsy).
- Laparoscopic cholecystectomy: prevents future events.

Gallstone pancreatitis

Stones in the *ampulla* or *pancreatic duct* that block the passage of pancreatic enzymes to the small intestines, resulting in a buildup of pancreatic enzymes, leading to pancreatic inflammation, and pancreatitis. This is the second most common cause of acute pancreatitis.

Diagnosis: CBC, electrolytes, liver enzymes, bilirubin, amylase/lipase (elevated), abdominal CT scan (identify pancreatitis), and ERCP (removes stone).

Treatment:

- Must be treated like any other pancreatitis with high fluid intake, narcotics (morphine), and bowel rest.
- ERCP with sphincterotomy (definitive treatment).

Ascending cholangitis

Medical emergency

Potentially fatal, acute bacterial infection (*E. coli* and other GI pathogens) of the biliary tree. Commonly caused by obstruction (choledocholithiasis).

Hx/PE:

- ➤ **Charcot's triad:** RUQ pain, jaundice, and fever.

- ➤ **Reynold's pentad:** Charcot's triad plus altered mental status and septic shock (hypotension).

Diagnosis:

- CBC (leukocytosis), CRP (elevated), ALT and AST levels (elevated), alkaline phosphatase level (high), bilirubin levels (high), lipase level (might be elevated), and blood culture (to rule out sepsis).

- First test is abdominal ultrasonography (to help distinguish between cholecystitis and ascending cholangitis).
- MRCP is a non-invasive test and has a sensitivity comparable to that of ERCP.
- Most accurate diagnostic test and treatment is ERCP.

Note: ERCP is the cause of acute pancreatitis in 5% of the cases. After the procedure, it can take a while for the levels of bilirubin, lipase, and alkaline phosphates to normalize. These studies can be repeated in a few weeks to check for normalization.

Treatment:

- ICU admission, IV hydration, blood pressure support, and IV antibiotics (ceftriaxone and metronidazole).
- Emergency ERCP is the treatment of choice (for bile duct decompression).
- Cholecystectomy.
- In severe cases, perform drainage and open decompression.
- Sphincterotomy: can be delayed for 72 hours after starting antibiotics or until fever subsides.

Mirizzi syndrome

Mirizzi syndrome (rare) is a type of obstructive jaundice that occurs when a large *cystic duct* stone compresses the adjacent common bile duct or hepatic duct, causing obstruction and jaundice. It can be associated with ascending cholangitis.

Diagnosis:

- Order common biliary laboratory tests, ultrasonography, abdominal CT scan, and MRCP (diagnostic).
- Can use ERCP for an existing ascending cholangitis.

Treatment: Laparoscopic cholecystectomy.

Gallstone ileus

Rare case of small bowel obstruction caused by a large gallstone stone (>2.5 cm) passing into the lumen of the small intestines via a cholecystoduodenal fistula.

Hx/PE: Similar to small bowel obstruction with recurrent dull pain, hyperactive bowel sounds, and distended abdomen.

Diagnosis:

- Abdominal radiography: "pneumobilia gas" in the biliary tree with possible multiple distended loops of the small bowel.
- Abdominal CT scan can be performed to confirm the diagnosis.

Treatment: **Laparotomy enterolithotomy.**

Primary sclerosing cholangitis (PSC)

Thought to be an autoimmune disorder that causes inflammation, fibrosis, and strictures of the intra and extra-hepatic bile ducts. Inflammation and fibrosis leads to obstruction and buildup of bile acids, which cause liver disease and cancer.

Risk factors: ulcerative colitis (80%), Crohn's disease, and polyarteritis nodosa (PAN).

Hx/PE: Progressive jaundice, pruritus, fat-soluble vitamin malabsorption, steatorrhea, and fatigue.

Diagnosis:

- Order: alkaline phosphatase level (high), liver enzymes (high) and bilirubin levels.
- Positivity for P-ANCA (30–80% [not specific]).
- MRCP/ERCP (multiple bile duct strictures and dilations "beading").
- Biopsy: periductal sclerosis (onion skinning).

Treatment: High-dose ursodeoxycholic acid, ERCP (dilation and stenting of strictures). Vitamin D, E, C, and K replacement, and liver transplant (definitive treatment).

Note: PSC has an increased risk of **cholangiocarcinoma**.

Primary biliary cirrhosis (PBC)

An autoimmune disorder more common in middle-aged women, causing destruction of the intrahepatic bile ducts of the liver, resulting in bile obstruction. The bile causes inflammation, fibrosis, and destruction of liver tissues <u>leading</u> to cirrhosis and end-stage liver disease.

Hx/PE: Malabsorption (fat-soluble vitamins), jaundice (elevated bilirubin), and pruritus (elevated bilirubin).

Diagnosis:

- Initial tests: AST and ALT levels (elevated), alkaline phosphatase level (high), and bilirubin levels (high).
- Ultrasonography and HIDA scan must be performed to rule out other sources of obstruction.
  - Consider abdominal CT scan and abdominal MRI.
- Most accurate tests are **anti-mitochondrial antibody** and liver biopsy.
- ERCP can be helpful in confirming diagnosis but not always performed.

Treatment:

- **Ursodeoxycholic acid:** can decrease progression of disease and help increase the rate of transport of bile acids and dissolve small stones.
  - A good alternative for patients who refuse surgery or are not eligible candidates for surgery.
- **Cholestyramine** (bile acid sequestrant): drug of choice for <u>pruritus</u> and effective against <u>diarrhea</u>.
- Steroids are <u>not</u> useful, despite being an autoimmune disease.
- Liver transplant is a definitive treatment. Bilirubin levels are considered predictive for the procedure.
- Supplement fat-soluble vitamins.

Note: Should separate dosage of ursodeoxycholic acid and cholestyramine by at least 2 hours, since cholestyramine interferes with absorption of ursodeoxycholic acid.

Porcelain gallbladder

The direct cause of this condition is unknown, but associated with chronic or excessive gallstones and strongly associated with gallbladder cancer.

Diagnosis: Abdominal ultrasonography or abdominal CT scan. Radiological studies show "calcification of the gallbladder."

Treatment: Elective laparoscopic cholecystectomy.

Note: Biopsy is not required for porcelain gallbladder.

Cholangiocarcinoma

Arises from the epithelial cells of the bile ducts. The prognosis is usually poor because detected late. It can be associated with PSC and *Clonorchis sinensis*.

Hx/PE: "Painless jaundice," weight loss, and fever.

Diagnosis:

- Order: liver enzyme (elevated), alkaline phosphate (elevated), and bilirubin levels (elevated).
- Ultrasonography, abdominal CT scan, and ERCP (biopsy).

Treatment: Surgical extraction, palliative chemotherapy (usually found in late stages), with or without radiation.

Liver diseases

Hepatitis

Inflammation of the liver, which leads to cell injury, fibrosis, and necrosis. Evidence of coagulopathy or encephalopathy can be signs of poor prognosis of liver disease.

Risk factors: alcohol, viruses, toxins, and medications (NSAIDs).

Hx/PE: Acute: flu-like symptoms followed by jaundice and RUQ tenderness.

Diagnosis:

- Laboratory tests: LFT levels (elevated), albumin level (low), bilirubin levels (elevated), PTT (elevated later stages), PT (elevated later stages), platelet count (low), bleeding time (elevated), alkaline phosphatase level (elevated), serum ammonia level (elevated later stages) viral hepatitis serology, and imaging studies (hematomegalia).

  - Viral hepatitis (ALT > AST).
  - Alcohol hepatitis (AST > ALT).

- In case of <u>chronic</u> or <u>severe</u> disease, a liver biopsy must be considered (to determine damage to the liver).

Note: MELD score includes creatinine, bilirubin, and INR.

Special tests:

➢ **Hemochromatosis** (iron studies and HFe mutation).

➢ **Wilson's disease** (ceruloplasmin and slit lamp).

➢ **Autoimmune hepatitis** (ANA, anti-smooth muscle antibody, and Coombs test).

➢ **Primary biliary cirrhosis** (anti-mitochondrial antibody and liver biopsy).

➢ **PSC** (p-ANCA [not very specific]).

➢ **Alcohol hepatitis** (AST > ALT).

➢ **Viral hepatitis** (ALT > AST).

Note: Mallory bodies are highly suggestive of alcohol hepatitis.

Treatment:

- Severe alcohol hepatitis (steroids).
- Autoimmune hepatitis (steroids and azathioprine).
- HBV (if symptomatic, IFN-α and lamivudine).
- HCV (if symptomatic, IFN-α and ribavirin).
- End-stage liver disease (transplant).

Note: Alcoholics who need a liver transplant will usually be required to join a rehabilitation center while on the waiting list and refrain from alcohol consumption for at least 6 months.

Viral hepatitis

Types (A, B, C, D, E):

- ➤ IgM HAVAb (observed in acute hepatitis A).
- ➤ IgG HAVAb (observed weeks-months later and a marker of previous infection).
- ➤ IgM anti-HBc (usually appears early in the clinical phase).
- ➤ IgG anti-HBc (appears weeks later).
- ➤ HBsAg (first marker detected and found in the carrier state).
- ➤ HBsAb (immunity or vaccination).
- ➤ HBcAg (core antigen).
- ➤ HBcAb (observed in the window period).
- ➤ HBeAg (indicates transmissibility).
- ➤ HBeAb (indicates low transmissibility).
- ➤ Hepatitis E (pregnant patients have a 20% mortality rate owing to **fulminant hepatic failure**).

Hepatitis C virus

Can be contracted via IV drug use, transfusion, needle-stick injury, and sexual contact.

Diagnosis:

- Laboratory levels depend on stage: hepatitis serology, liver enzyme levels, bilirubin, alkaline phosphatase, PT/INR, PTT, bleeding time, albumin, ammonia, and platelet count.
- HCV RNA has a high specificity.
- Patients with advanced disease will require a liver biopsy to determine whether a liver transplant will be necessary.

Treatment:

- If asymptomatic, supportive measures are sufficient.
- Treatment with pegylated-interferon (INF-α) <u>plus</u> **ribavirin**; can be started when the patient is symptomatic or exhibits symptoms of liver disease.
  - If elevated AST and moderate inflammation on liver biopsy consider treatment.

- Genotype 1 can be treated with **ledipasvir** and **sofosbuvir** with a cure rate of 95%.

Note: Interferon can cause thrombocytopenia and flu-like symptoms.

Prevention:

➤ Vaccination against hepatitis A and B.

➤ No vaccine available against hepatitis C.

Hepatitis B virus

Commonly transferred via sexual intercourse, IV needles, and blood transfusions. Only 5% of adult patients show progression to chronic disease. Hepatitis B is <u>not</u> a contraindication for breastfeeding.

Diagnosis:

- Laboratory tests: CBC (monitor platelets), liver enzymes, bilirubin, alkaline phosphate, PT/INR, PTT, platelets, bleeding time, serum ammonia, albumin, and hepatitis serology.

- Liver imagining and biopsy are needed for chronic and advanced disease.

Treatment:

- Most patients can be managed with supportive measures.

- IFN-α and **lamivudine** can be administered if the condition is severe, concurrent hepatitis C, immunosuppressed, or the patient is symptomatic.

Prevention:

- If a <u>non</u>-immune individual (HBsAb negative) sustains a needle-stick injury with a needle used by an infected individual, then both hepatitis B vaccination <u>and</u> HBIG can be administered .

- Update hepatitis B and A vaccinations.

Budd-Chiari syndrome

Extremely rare condition characterized by thrombosis of the hepatic <u>veins</u>. These veins drain the liver and when obstructed cause hepatic out flow obstruction. The risk factors are the same as those for thrombosis.

Hx/PE: <u>Triad</u>: chronic vague abdominal pain, hepatomegaly, and ascites.

Diagnosis: LFTs (levels elevated) and most common diagnostic methods are ultrasonography and retrograde angiography.

Treatment:

- Anti-coagulation medication (heparin to warfarin bridge).
- Ascites: low-salt diet and diuretics.
- If develop fulminant liver failure may require liver transplant.

Hepatocellular carcinoma

The most common liver cancer caused by a variety of pathologies. The prognosis will depend on tumor size, staging, and grading.

Risk factors: cirrhosis (most common cause in the United States), HBV (most common cause in China) HCV, aflatoxins, Wilson's disease, α-1 antitrypsin, and hemochromatosis.

Hx/PE: RUQ abdominal pain, jaundice, edema, ascites, weight loss, abdominal distention, easy bruisability, AMS, and coagulopathy.

Diagnosis:

- Order: CBC, albumin level (low), PT/INR (elevated), PTT (elevated), LFTs (levels elevated), serum ammonia, hepatitis serology, and **α-fetoprotein levels** (levels can correspond to tumor size).
- The first radiological test is abdominal ultrasonography (which is also cost effective) and often used for surveillance.
- In case of elevated levels of α-fetoprotein, the best diagnostic test is abdominal CT scan with contrast.
- Liver biopsy (definitive) is not always needed, if distinct patterns are seen on abdominal CT scan.

Note: Alpha-1 antitrypsin deficiency is a genetic disorder that can cause hepatocellular carcinoma and panacinar emphysema.

Treatment:

- Chemotherapy and radiation (are not very helpful but can shrink the tumor prior to surgery).
- Tumor resection or liver transplantation.
- Monitor tumor by serial α-fetoprotein levels.

Prevention: vaccination against hepatitis B and hepatitis A. Decrease alcohol intake.

Hepatic adenomas

A rare, benign hepatic tumor in women aged 20 to 40 years, common among those who use oral contraceptives (with high levels of estrogen) or anabolic steroids. If large, they are prone to rupture and hemorrhages.

Diagnosis: Abdominal ultrasound followed by abdominal CT scan or MRI (most specific test).

Treatment:

- If not ruptured and small (<5 cm), OCP or steroids can be stopped and the adenoma usually regresses spontaneously. Monitor via radiological studies and α-fetoprotein levels.
- In case of rupture or large (>5 cm), emergency surgery will be considered.

Hemochromatosis

Hyperabsorption or accumulation of iron in the body and elevated hemosiderin levels that can deposit in various organs.

Types:

➤ Primary hemochromatosis: (AR), genetic testing for C282Y mutation on the HFE gene, which is more common in males.

➤ Secondary hemochromatosis: caused by hemolytic anemia or blood transfusions.

Hx/PE: Abdominal pain, "bronze skin pigmentation," hypogonadism, diabetes, arthropathy of MCP joints, heart failure (restrictive cardiomyopathy), and cirrhosis.

Diagnosis:

- Best initial test is **fasting transferrin saturation** (>45%) (most sensitive test) and iron studies (increased serum iron, increased ferritin, and decreased TIBC).
- Glucose intolerance with mildly elevated liver enzyme and alkaline phosphatase level.

- **HFe gene mutation** (most specific test for primary hemochromatosis).
- Most accurate test is liver biopsy (hepatic iron index).
  - Can avoid liver biopsy in case of positive MRI result and HFe gene mutation.

Treatment:

- Primary disease: weekly **phlebotomy** until iron levels decrease or normalize. Then maintenance phlebotomies at least every 2-4 months.

- Secondary disease: in case of iron overload, first-line treatment is **deferoxamine**.

Note: All symptomatic patients must undergo a phlebotomy unless contraindicated.

Wilson's disease (hepatolenticular degeneration)

Autosomal recessive-mutation in the *Wilson disease protein gene* on chromosome 13, which causes abnormal copper accumulation mainly in the liver and the brain.

Hx/PE: "**ABCD**": **a**sterixis, **b**asal ganglion (Parkinson-like), **c**irrhosis, **Kayser-Fleischer rings,** and **d**ementia.

Diagnosis:

- First conduct the slit-lamp test (sensitive test), followed by **ceruloplasmin test** (decreased).

  - Low serum ceruloplasmin concentration (<0.2 g/L) and evidence of Keyser-Fleischer rings on the slit-lamp.

- Order: ALT (elevated), AST (elevated), alkaline phosphate (elevated), and bilirubin levels (elevated).

- Copper in the urine and liver (elevated).

- Most accurate test is liver biopsy (elevated copper) and genetic testing.

Note: If signs of portal hypertension are observed, esophageal varices must be ruled out by upper endoscopy.

- **Penicillamine** (first line treatment) a copper chelator + pyridoxine (B6).
- Long-term prevention is copper restriction (seafood, nuts, mushrooms, and liver ingestion).
- Liver transplant (effective cure).

Note: Penicillamine can cause aplastic anemia.

Cirrhosis

Fibrosis and nodular regeneration caused by chronic hepatocellular injury.

<u>Risk factors</u>: alcohol (most common cause), chronic viral hepatitis, primary biliary cirrhosis, α-1 antitrypsin deficiency, medications, and Budd-Chiari syndrome.

Hx/PE: Jaundice, edema, ascites (transudate SAAG >1.1 g/dL), SBP, hepatic encephalopathy, palmar erythema, gynecomastia, gastroesophageal varices, portal hypertension, coagulopathy, and renal dysfunction.

Diagnosis: Later finds for advanced cirrhosis: albumin (low), platelets (low), PT/INR (high), PTT (high), ammonium levels (high), ALT and AST (normal or low), bilirubin (high), and alkaline phosphatase.

Note: ALT and AST levels can be normal or low in patients with cirrhosis secondary to "hepatic burnout."

<u>Special laboratory tests</u>: viral hepatitis serology, iron studies, ceruloplasmin, α-1 antitrypsin, anti-smooth muscle antibody, and anti-mitochondrial antibody.

- Abdominal ultrasonography: monitor liver size, ascites, hepatic veins, and splenic veins.
- In the presence of ascites with new onset, pain, or fever; paracentesis must be conducted:
  - Measure SAAG = serum albumin − ascites albumin.
  - SAAG > 1.1 g/dL (transudate).
  - SAAG < 1.1 g/dL (exudative).

- Liver biopsy (fibrosis nodular regeneration) gold standard but not always needed.

Note: In elderly women with ascites, ovarian tumors must be ruled out with pelvic ultrasonography.

Treatment:

- Treat underlying causes.
- <u>Ascites</u>: restrict sodium, protein, and fluid intake.
    - If unresponsive to medications, perform serial taps (remove 2–4 L in case of good renal function).
- Diuretics must be started: furosemide and/or spironolactone.
- IV albumin for volume expansion of plasma.
- If caused by α-1 antitrypsin deficiency, then α-1 antitrypsin infusion will be required.

Note: Causes of transudate effusion (renal failure, heart failure, and liver failure), and require reduction of fluid, salt, and protein in the diet.

Spontaneous bacterial peritonitis (SBP)

This is an acute bacterial infection of the ascitic fluid and <u>almost</u> exclusively associated with portal hypertension. The most common etiological factor is infection with *E. coli*.

Hx/PE: If fever is present in patients with ascites then SBP should be suspected.

Diagnosis: Abdominal paracentesis culture: positive findings (i.e., >250 PMN or >500 WBC), blood culture studies will be necessary (to rule out sepsis).

Note: with Paracentesis order: Gram stain, LDH, glucose, albumin, proteins, and cell count.

Treatment:

- The patient must be hospitalized and started on IV antibiotics (ceftriaxone).
- IV albumin on day 1 and day 3 of hospitalization has been shown to decrease renal impairment.

- After discharge from the hospital, home prophylaxis can be maintained with levofloxacin (to decrease episodes).
- Also, give prophylactical fluoroquinolone for 7-10 days in patients with variceal bleeding.

Hepatorenal syndrome (HRS)

This is a life-threatening syndrome that consists of rapid deterioration of kidney function in individuals with hepatic dysfunction. Diagnosis is made by considering minor and major criteria (i.e., hepatic failure, portal hypertension, and renal failure <u>not</u> caused by other pathologies).

Hx/PE: AMS, oliguria, jaundice, and icterus.

Diagnosis:
- Complicated diagnosis of exclusion: LFTs and BUN/Cr ratio (elevated) to start suspicion.
- **Volume challenge test** should be obtained to rule out renal failure secondary to dehydration.

Treatment:
- Combination of octreotide and midodrine or norepinephrine, along with albumin can be helpful for volume expansion of plasma.
- Severe cases: dialysis and liver transplant.

Hepatic encephalopathy

This condition is observed in patients with a history of hepatitis or cirrhosis.

Hx/PE: Confusion and AMS.

Diagnosis: Serum ammonia levels (elevated), and history of liver disease.

Treatment:
- Restriction of proteins is <u>no</u> longer recommended for these patients, as adequate proteins and energy are needed.
- Branched-chain amino acids and probiotics are recommended.

- Lactulose and/or rifaximin are also helpful for removing ammonia.
- TIPS is contraindicated here, since it can worsen encephalopathy by bypassing the liver for detoxification.

Fun facts:

➤ Patients with AMS might require intubation and aspiration precautions.

➤ **Lactulose** (disaccharide) is not absorbed in the GI tract and causes a decrease in colonic pH, thus trapping ammonium ions and converting NH_3 to NH_4, which cannot be absorbed by the GI tract.

➤ **Rifaximin** works by maintaining a low bacterial count in the GI tract, so that large amounts of ammonia waste products are not produced.

Pancreatic diseases

➤ Can be caused by ethanol (most common), gallstones, trauma, steroids, mumps, scorpion stings, hypercalcemia, hyperlipidemia (triglycerides > 1,000 mg/dL), and drugs ("GET SMASHED").

➤ Triglycerides can artificially reduce amylase and lipase levels, so the condition becomes harder to diagnose.

Note: If not caused by gallstones or ethanol, then hypercalcemia is the next common cause.

Acute pancreatitis

Commonly caused by gallstones and ethanol.

Complications:

➤ Recurrent acute pancreatitis → Can lead to chronic pancreatitis.

➤ Pancreatic pseudocyst → No leukocytosis or fever.

➤ Necrotizing pancreatitis → Leukocytosis and high fever.

➤ Pancreatic abscess → Leukocytosis and fever.

- Pancreatic cancer → Painless jaundice with weight loss.
- ARDS (life-threatening complication of acute pancreatitis); can cause alveolar capillary membrane destruction because of the circulating phospholipase.

Hx/PE: Severe epigastric pain radiating to the back (worsens when lying down), flatulence, steatorrhea, Grey Turner's sign (flank discoloration), and Cullen's sign (periumbilical discoloration). Tenderness on epigastric palpation.

Diagnosis:

- Best initial test: amylase (sensitive) and/or lipase (specific) levels.
- Abdominal radiography and serum calcium level (decreased), "soap bubbles."
- Most accurate test: abdominal CT scan (specific 85%).
  - Abdominal CT scan: Can detect pancreatic necrosis.

Note: APACHE score can be used to determine the severity of pancreatitis and does not need 48 hours of hospitalization like the previously used Ranson criteria.

Treatment:

- NPO, NG-tube, high fluid intake (first step), and high-dose analgesia.
- Decrease alcohol and fat intake.

Note: Check for signs of necrotizing pancreatitis or pancreatic abscess (leukocytosis and fever).

Chronic pancreatitis

Commonly caused by alcohol (90%) and multiple episodes of pancreatitis.

Diagnosis:

- Elevated amylase and lipase (normal or high) production caused by "pancreatic burn out."
  - Amylase and lipase level not very effective for diagnosis of

chronic pancreatitis.

- Best initial test: abdominal radiography (may see calcifications) and abdominal CT scan w/o contrast.

- Most accurate test: **secretin stimulation test** (90% specific), which in a normal healthy pancreas will result in a large amount of bicarbonate but not in chronic pancreatitis.

Note: Chronic pancreatitis: best initial radiological test is abdominal radiography and abdominal CT scan, followed by secretin stimulation test, which is the most accurate test for chronic pancreatitis.

Treatment:

- NPO, NG-tube, high fluid intake, analgesics, exogenous lipase, amylase, trypsin, medium-chain fatty acid, low-fat diet, vitamins, and celiac nerve block (last resort).

- Give pancreatic enzymes with omeprazole to protect from GI acids.

Note: In case of pancreatic necrosis, first perform pancreatic aspiration of that tissue. If aspiration shows infection, then surgical debridement and antibiotics (imipenem) are indicated and blood culture must be performed.

Pancreatic pseudocysts

Pancreatic fluids rich in pancreatic enzymes that typically collect in the lesser sac of the abdomen. They can be self-limiting and can cause impingement on nearby structures. They can be secondary to trauma or a complication of pancreatitis.

Diagnosis:

- No fever or leukocytosis.

- Lipase, amylase, and abdominal CT scan (gold standard).

Treatment:

- If patient is symptomatic (pain) or shows signs of infection (fever), drainage must be considered.
  - If the cyst is painful, >6 cm, or the condition has been present for >6 weeks, perform drainage.
  - If the condition is painless and small, drainage is not required.

Pancreatic cancer

Adenocarcinoma in 75% of the cases, common in the pancreatic head, "painless progressive obstructive jaundice."

Risk factors: chronic pancreatitis, alcohol, smoking, and high-fat diet.

Hx/PE: Weight loss, Courvoisier's sign (palpable non-tender gallbladder), and no abdominal pain radiating to the back.

Diagnosis:
- First initial test is abdominal CT scan and measure CA-19-9 level (elevated).
- ERCP (highly sensitive) can be performed for biopsy.
- If a tumor is present at the pancreatic head, it might show distal common bile duct narrowing.

Note: Trousseau's sign: spontaneous recurrent thrombosis (**migratory thrombophlebitis**) caused by decreased calcium levels.

Treatment:

The only possible curable treatment is surgical intervention with **Whipple's procedure** (pancreaticoduodenectomy).

- In case of metastatic disease, consider palliative care (death in 6 months).

Index

A

acalculous cholecystitis 42
achalasia 6
alcohol hepatitis 50
alpha-1 antitrypsin deficiency 53
alpha-fetoprotein levels 53
amebic 18
anti-intrinsic factor antibodies 13
anti-mitochondrial antibody 48
anti-parietal cell antibodies 13
APACHE score 60
ascending cholangitis 45
autoimmune hepatitis 50

B

bacillus cereus 18
Barrett's esophagus 8

C

campylobacter 17, 19
candida albicans 11
carcinoid syndrome 24
ceruloplasmin test 55
Charcot's triad 45
cholangiocarcinoma 47, 49
cholecystitis 42
cholecystoduodenal fistula 47
choledocholithiasis 44
cholescintigraphy 42
cholestyramine 44, 48
clostridium difficile 19
clostridium perfringens 18
colorectal cancer 33
colovesical fistula 41
Crohn's disease 39
cryptosporidium 18
cytomegalovirus 12

D

deferoxamine 55
diarrhea 16
diltiazem 4
diverticulosis 30
dumping syndrome 16, 28

E

echinococcus 22
entamoeba histolytica 20
epiphrenic diverticulum 5
escherichia coli o157h7 20
esophageal cancer 7
esophageal diverticula 5
esophageal dysphagia 2
esophageal motility study 4
esophageal perforation 11
esophageal spasm 4
esophageal varices 9
esophageal webs 3

F

familial adenomatous polyposis 35
fasting transferrin saturation 54
fistula-in-ano 41
fistulotomy 41
fulminant hepatic failure 51

G

gallstone ileus 47
gallstone pancreatitis 45
Gardner's syndrome 35
gastric adenocarcinoma with
    Krukenberg tumor 36
gastric cancer 13
gastric emptying study 27
gastritis 12

Index, continued

gastrograffin contrast esophagram 11

giardia lamblia 17

H

hemochromatosis 50, 54
hemorrhoids 32, 33
hepatic adenomas 54
hepatic encephalopathy 58
hepatic iminodiacetic acid level 42
hepatitis 49
hepatitis, viral 51
hepatocellular carcinoma 53
hepatolenticular degeneration 55
hepatorenal syndrome 58
hereditary nonpolyposis colorectal cancer 35
herpes simplex virus 12
Hesselbach's triangle 40
HFE gene mutation 55
hiatal hernias 9
hookworms 22
hydrogen breath test 23

I

inguinal hernias 40
irritable bowel syndrome 24

K

Kayser-Fleischer rings 55

L

lactose intolerance 23
lactulose 59
lamivudine 52
laparoscopic appendectomy 32
laparoscopic cholecystectomy 43
laparotomy enterolithotomy 47
large bowel obstruction 26
ledipasvir 52

leukoplakia 11
lower GI bleeding 37
Lynch syndrome 35

M

malabsorption 23
Mallory-Weiss 10
malt lymphoma 35
MELD score 50
mesenteric angiography 29
mesenteric ischemia 29
migratory thrombophlebitis 62

N

Nissen fundoplication 7
non-caseating granulomas 39
nutcracker esophagus 4

O

Ogilvie syndrome 27
oropharyngeal dysphagia 2

P

pancreatic cancer 62
pancreatic necrosis 61
pancreatic pseudocysts 61
pancreatitis 59, 60
paraesophageal hiatal hernias 9
penicillamine 56
peptic ulcer disease 15
Peutz-Jeghers syndrome 34
phlebotomy 55
pinworms 22
porcelain gallbladder 49
primary biliary cirrhosis 48, 50
primary sclerosing cholangitis 47, 50
Prinzmetal's angina 4
pseudomembranous 19

Index, continued

R

Ranson criteria 60
Reynold's pentad 45
ribavirin 51
rifaximin 59
roundworm 22
rubber band ligation 33

S

salmonella 21
salmonellosis enteritidis 18
sclerotherapy 33
secretin stimulation test 14, 61
shigella 21
sliding hiatal hernias 9
small bowel obstruction 25
sofosbuvir 52
spontaneous bacterial peritonitis 57
staphylococcus aureus 17
stones 44
Sudan black stain 23
surgical gastropexy 9

T

total proctocolectomy 35, 38
toxic megacolon 38
traction diverticulum 5
transjugular intrahepatic portosystemic shunt 10
Turcot syndrome 35

U

ulcerative colitis 37
upper GI bleeding 36
ursodeoxycholic acid 44, 48

V

vibrio parahaemolyticus 17

video pill endoscopy 14
viral hepatitis 50
volume challenge test 58

W

Whipple disease 18
Whipple's procedure 62
Wilson's disease 50, 55

Y

yersinia enterocolitica 22

Z

Zenker's diverticulum 5
Zollinger-Ellison syndrome 14